UNTIL IT FEELS RIGHT

Emily Costa

autofocus books
Orlando, Florida

Published by Autofocus Books
PO Box 560002
Orlando, Fl 32856
autofocuslit.com

Memoir/Diary
ISBN: 978-1-957392-05-9

Cover Illustrations ©Amy Wheaton
Library of Congress Control Number: 2022937220

For my enablers

UNTIL IT FEELS RIGHT

1998-1999

This thing starts in sixth grade. A teenager working for my dad—a friend of the family, a one-time babysitter—bludgeons a kid my age. It's like okay, sure, I've always thought of death death death, even as a toddler, ever since watching my grandfather wither from cancer and hallucinate in our TV room recliner, but it's like *bam*, now every thought flips to murder, to quick death, bloody death, a sledgehammer to the head, and this little part of my brain, this tiny voice says *but—and hear me out—what if you could predict death? What if you could predict murder?* and the rest of my brain says *I'm listening*, so I stop feeling my body for tumors all the time and start becoming aware of shadows, of branch-snaps, of suspicious-looking men. I'm afraid of being alone outside. And then, inside. The little part of my brain, which is really the main part of my brain even though its voice starts out so weak, says *well wouldn't you want to do anything and everything in your power to avoid the murder then?* To which the rest of my brain says *duh*, and the little part goes on saying *so how do you know there's no one hiding in your closet?* And I realize I don't know that, I have no clue, and it says *so do you... maybe wanna check in there?* Then my body checks, rushes over to push back clothes, to peek into the black spaces, and the little part of my brain says *you know a person could fit under a bed too*, and the rest of me says *ah yes true*, so I check, and the little part of my brain likes this and says *well potentially a person could fit behind your door...and definitely behind your curtains, maybe balancing on the baseboard heater to hide their feet...and maybe a really small person could fold up and fit into your drawers, or they've carved out the inside of your dresser completely while you were at school and they're living in there, waiting to pounce*, and that tiny part loves it because the rest of me is pure fear. And fear beats reality every single time.

But all of this still makes some sense, even as the ritual crystallizes and forms an order. I walk clockwise around the room, door to dresser to closet to bed, back to door. I add in more precautions: I thumbtack an American flag over my closet doors as a kind of tamper-proof seal, since someone hiding in my closet wouldn't be able to replace the tacks after hiding inside. It slowly morphs from *do these things to make sure you are safe* to *do these things or else you will not be safe* to *do these things or else you will die.*

Then come the offshoots. The rational part of my brain still doesn't fully understand them, but luckily that other part tricks me into doing them anyway. It conjures horrifying bloody images played on loop. *This is you dead, Emily. This is you dead.* Sometimes the rest of me is feeling big, feeling brave, feeling tired, and I say *well fine, kill me, get it over with. This is hell.* And then the little part of my brain remembers the Columbine announcement on *Total Request Live*, the footage and interviews, the somber VJs. My brain flips through images, shows my mom shot at school while she's teaching. Her form fuzzy on security cam footage. Blood pooling. So I listen.

I am stuck on multiples of four. I like the balance of four, like legs supporting a tabletop, so I repeat everything four times. If I mess up within those four times, if I accidentally think of any of those bloody images on the last little tap-touch-count bit on the last run-through of the ritual, I have to restart, do it four more times. Sometimes I'm only able to get in two times if it happens in public. It's happening more in public.

The numbers, the counting—they're some kind of add-on. The nighttime rituals don't bring me enough comfort. It's like a drug, a little bit's good at first, but then it takes more and more just to feel normal, just to bring you back to yourself.

I wear the same pajamas to bed every night: white fleece dELiA*s pants with little blue stars on them that are probably my most prized possession because they were expensive, and a baby blue Paul Frank t-shirt with a turtle on it. During the day I hide them under my pillow, folded neatly, never washed.

Every part of my body holds meaning. My fingers

are coded: pointer is pointing—everyone will point and laugh at me; middle is fuck you, fuck like sex, sex like rape, rape and murder; ring finger like wring your neck.

Thumb and pinkie are fine. Thumb and pinkie are safe.

But I wouldn't, as I sit in bed in pajamas, comforter touching both of my hands with the same even pressure, describe the feeling as *safe*. It's blank. Exhausted. Sometimes the numbers go on forever. Sometimes I lose count. Then I sink into this space of fast repetition, so many times until it feels right—just *right*. I can't explain it any more than that. I never know when it'll feel right. I want to stick a needle into my ear canal and end all of it, end the part of me that won't quit.

2021

It's bad every day. I wake up, step out of bed, left foot right, softly, no flat slap on the floor, because if I have some violent movement right at the start, that means the day is fucked. I put on my pants, and then I take off my pants because I didn't have the right set of images and words in my head—I was picturing the faces of people close to me. I had the word *cancer* floating around. So I force in other images, ones of people I don't care about, neutral people, casual friends, minor acquaintances. I add in a neutral c-word. *Cold*, maybe. *Cupcake.* Sometimes I mouth it over and over so it's really stuck there, keeping the bad c-word away. I put on my pants again. I feel like one of those one-man bands, all my extremities focused and performing, and if the images keep forcing themselves in, it's pants off, pants on, pants off, pants on until I get it right. Then it's the shirt. And the socks. Walking through the doorway and fixing my hair and brushing my teeth. It's all day, and it doesn't stop. I'm talking to people, I'm teaching a college class. I'm making chicken nuggets, I'm playing Legos. I'm shaving my legs. I'm reading and re-reading. I'm in my head, and I'm touching only the things that feel right, and I'm avoiding, and I'm asking Jesse a million times *is it okay, are we going to die, are we going to get sick*, and I'm cleaning groceries and searching the internet and learning about death rates and percent-ages and one-in-eight women this, and how-many-days-from-exposure that. I'm washing and washing. If I keep doing these things the right way, the bad things I think about maybe won't happen. The *maybe* is the thing. I know what I do doesn't change shit. I'm not living to-tally in delusion. I'm not fucking stupid, or that stupid. But what if it does? Just in case, I better do it. I did these rituals so the cancer wouldn't kill my dad, and he died in January. But what if I made him last a little longer? What if it would have been worse if I didn't do this? What if I was staving off some other unknown fate, like my mom dying, or Jesse dying, or my kid dying? Every so often my psychiatrist will draw a picture on a sheet of blank white paper. A little dot. *That's you*, he says. *You're a speck.* And then a big big circle around it. *That's the universe. You don't control any of it.*

A month ago, I found a lump on my right breast. I'd just found a tumor on my dog, his lymph node, a bulge on the back of his thigh. I started spiraling. I couldn't sleep. I was picturing what I'd look like bald, planning out who could help Jesse raise Ezra. Because I was dead. For sure. I was walking around crying and dry-heaving, and I was stuck outside doorways because

I was too overwhelmed to do a clean, perfect ritual. I couldn't get into rooms. In out, in out. I'd press my fingers into my closed eyelids until I saw blurred electric shapes in the black. Some days I couldn't even get in the house. I made a promise to whoever, maybe to myself, that if it wasn't cancer, I'd give it one final go, really try to get rid of it. I'd tried everything, I thought.

I told my mom what I was thinking and she texted me a link to a hospital a half hour away. I scrolled and found it: an outpatient program for cognitive behavioral therapy, a really intensive one, where for two hours every weekday for three weeks I would be forced to confront situations that scare me and try to change the ways I respond to them. *Thank you*, I texted. Sometimes instead of talking things through to come up with an answer, she'll google and send a link. She wants things fixed. I suspect, too, she didn't want to deal with my bullshit anymore, years and years of this. She'd brought me to a hospital before, the Yale one, adolescent unit. I tried to die when I was fifteen.

At my intake for CBT, my clinician, C, had me go over that hospital stay, the assault that happened a few months before it, this and all the bad stuff in my life, the bouts of depression, the self-harm, the medications. That two-month period last winter where I had to get drunk every night to fall sleep. He was kind and calm and made it easy for me to go on. Three hours of it. Every traumatic thing. Every ritual laid out. *You've been just white-knuckling it, haven't you*, he said.

Monday, October 4, 2021

Drove all the way to Hartford, got stuck in traffic, couldn't find the right parking lot. Exactly what I thought would happen. More proof it's going to be difficult to break the causal link between my thoughts and these negative outcomes. Called C twice and he was super nice about it. The place is through a little courtyard. Rain all day. I'd been listening to Cake the whole way there. I really love *Fashion Nugget*. I had the CD when I was fourteen but who knows what I did with it. The songs were all familiar which made me less anxious when I was driving in the rain doing eighty, a very dangerous thing I realize now that I type it out.

When I got to his office, C asked me some questions about suicide, which I think they have to ask every time. I'm not suicidal right now. We talked a little about CBT and what we'd be doing. I've done it twice before, but I was young and stupid and didn't want to put in any effort to get better, so I mostly lied that I'd been practicing. Plus I only saw those doctors once a week. C made this really great list on the whiteboard of my thoughts, rituals, fears, things like that. I don't remember the categories because it just looks like I'm fucking insane when it's all written out, and I kept being like *oh, also this, also that*—all the random rituals and shit I do that were just coming into my head. He told me it's about breaking down these links, to sever the ties between thought and action and consequence and something else. Like retrain my brain. We came up with a list of exposures that might be good to try, and it was a pretty long list, and at first I was nervous because I didn't think I'd be good at coming up with ideas but turns out I am because it's just the opposite of what I'd want to do. *Hmm what's the scariest thing? Oh let's do that.*

The first thing was I had to say the word cancer for a full five minutes straight, which wasn't as hard or scary as I thought it was going to be, and mostly the word just sounded bizarre and I kept almost laughing, but he was doing it too, which helped. I focused solely on making sure I said the word and wondering how much time had passed. I started getting nervous I'd say some other word, which was distracting, but maybe it was good I was thinking and being anxious about that instead of the idea that by saying cancer I was somehow manifesting the disease into me, into my family. We made it harder by saying it for another five minutes (which is longer than it sounds), but this time I held my phone while doing it. The background is a picture of my dad and my brother and Ezra, so that put some thoughts in my head. Bad ones. My dad in hospice. I was still anxious at the end, but it wasn't the really high number I reported at the beginning, which was probably in the eighties or nineties.

I felt exhausted when I got home. At night, I did the homework: say *cancer* again while holding my phone for five to fifteen minutes. I was only able to do five. I felt like it was harder to do it at home. I kept seeing those pictures of my dad on my phone and then pictures of deathbed stuff kept coming into my head—the way his eyes moved or didn't, that fixed eye thing right before you die, that waxy skin, the sunken-in face.

Tuesday, October 5, 2021

I taught today and at school I'm high anxiety the whole fucking time. Trying to focus on what I'm saying while watching all of them adjust their masks, cough, use their phones. We were in the library learning how to do research which every year is in this huge room, so I was like *sweet, there will actually be some air flow*, but instead we were in this other room that was half the size of our normal classroom. And right before we went there, I walked by the girl who always has her nose out of her mask, and her back was to me, and she sucked in a massive amount of snot because she's in class even though she's been sick for many weeks and I know, despite my suggestion and reporting her, that she hasn't tested, she's still in class. I sound so lame, such a fucking snitch, but I'm scared. I turned as I walked away from her, and her whole mask was OFF. I was ready to tap out for the day. The girl who had the negative test was there, and I should be fine around her since she said it was negative, but still I was like *hmm do I believe you?*

So after class I asked her two more times and she probably thought I was crazy. C calls this "reassurance-seeking," which I do a lot. But there were other people sniffling and I had to be close to them and I hated it. I tried to just stay in the doorway. The librarian teacher was super close to them the whole time and to me too, so I started to think maybe that's the normal thing to do, because she's one of the smartest people I've ever met. If she was okay with it, it must be fine. And this is what I do—I'm constantly comparing my behavior to other people's because I've totally lost any sense of rationality. While the students worked, she told me a story about how one of her students was always absent because his dog was dying, how he said he has to be near the dog to make sure she's okay during surgery. She wanted to tell him that he can't do anything while the dog's in surgery so he might as well come to class, and then she said *I thought, wow, that's probably the hardest thing he ever had to go through,* but she said it kind of like, or I took it as, *life will get so much harder.* And I said *oh that's sad, my dog has cancer, it can be rough,* and she was like *aww,* and I said *yeah and my dad died a few months ago* and kind of laughed like *crazy times, right.* I guess I was trying to say you can have legit bad shit in your life and a dying dog is still very bad. I felt suddenly and oddly protective of this kid. Maybe because I was thinking this kid could very well be me. Then I said *this year sucks,* and she agreed. Most people agree. I don't know why I felt the need to type that. But I did get a really good parking spot and was early and could leave right on time, which was something I'd been worrying about that morning.

I did a virtual session with C when I got home. We did so much. I still can't believe it. We did the cancer thing again to reinforce it, and then I said *cancer* while plugging in my phone, and when I did, it DIDN'T CHARGE, which freaked me out. I paused the exposure to tell him, and then I started noticing the numbers on my phone and oh man, when I start noticing numbers I get nuts. This will be the age, date, whatever, that I'll die. I told him about that because it's in my best interest to say these things even if they will make me have to do a hard exposure. That's obviously what happened. He told me to pick an age, and so I picked thirty-seven, which is a few years away, and I had to repeat *I will die when I'm thirty-seven* for five straight minutes. All my muscles were tight and I was at like a ninety-five on the anxiety scale at one point and then the sentences blurred and my mouth was dry. It's scary to even type that. I told my family later, and they were like *holy shit I couldn't do any of that*, which made me feel accomplished but also like, yeah, I hate that I said it too. But I said it so much that I can't undo it. I'm just kind of sitting here and can't move. Because what happens is that I start to believe I'm infecting the future, or I'm creating a future where this will happen. So then we got my shoes and I showed him that I was putting them on as I said *cancer* and *COVID*, and it wasn't that bad because I knew I'd take them off within a few minutes, like I wouldn't be contaminating/changing too much of the future. I told him this and he told me to put them on again and say *I will get in a car accident* and go take a drive, and I laughed, but he was serious, and I said *okay, I'll take a picture to prove it* but he said he believes me. So I did that, and I was freaked out turning onto the main road, but I came back smiling. But then I stopped smiling because I felt like maybe I cheated death. I have to try it again when I'm going to pick up Ezra or something.

The next thing I did was empty out all the packages of masks that have been sitting on my dining room table for a month to "cool off." My hands felt filthy and disgusting but I stuck with it. And I couldn't wash them after at all. Which, yikes! During this whole thing Angus was ripping apart the recycling. I'm embarrassed of the state of my house, so I was pretty careful about C not seeing it as I carried around the laptop, but I felt like a revolting person during this whole part of my session. But I did it. Then he even clapped at two parts and said I was doing a good job. I'm such a suck-up teacher's pet and that's what I need. My homework after was to, before bed, plug in my phone while saying cancer and leave it plugged the whole night after doing it just once, and then in the morning to put on clothes and shoes while saying *cancer* or *COVID*, and do it JUST ONCE, which is extremely difficult for me because ideally it should be four perfect times, or at least an even number.

I did a lot of terrifying things today. I'm proud I guess.

Wednesday, October 6, 2021

Today I did a virtual session. I was okay doing the little homework I had—plugging in my phone once while saying *cancer*. Getting dressed doing the same thing. But the big issue was that I woke up with a sore throat. Ezra has been sick for a week with sinus congestion (I'm usually not too insane if there's only this symptom and no additional symptoms) and I'd been fighting it off, taking Emergen-C, but I guess it caught up to me. But because I had the sore throat, which he didn't have, I freaked. I tried to take a rapid test but couldn't find one, so I bought an at-home kit which, in the past, I was not confident about, but because I had symptoms I think it was okay. It was negative thankfully. I was a little nauseated and shaky waiting the fifteen minutes. I emailed C, and it was okay to do a virtual session. My COVID anxiety was high, but not as high as I thought it'd be because it wasn't the unknown of an exposure. It was like *well, this is probably a cold, I've seen how it moves.* I had this great idea of going to the grocery store beforehand and getting some stuff so that I could eventually put it away without cleaning it. Typing that, I'm realizing it's shitty to go out while sick, but hopefully my constant hand-washing and mask-wearing cancel that out. But I got all the groceries and placed them in the cart thinking about how they'd end up in my pantry and fridge unclean. Why am I torturing myself, why am I coming up with GREAT IDEAS to torture myself, but I know I have to be honest and do it.

So first we worked on some reinforcing stuff, cancer and the phone, the *I will die when I'm thirty-seven* stuff again, but I started thinking that maybe thirty-seven was too far in the future, so although it is extremely anxiety-inducing and scary, maybe I should pick some day closer to present, and he said *you can say you're gonna die like in five minutes*, and I was like *holy shit*, and so we did an exposure where I was like *I'm going to die at 2:38 on October 6, 2021* and we started two minutes before that, and the anxiety crested in much the way you'd think, peaking during that minute I said I was going to die, but then I didn't die (although I hate typing that out for some reason again, like I'm cheating death and will pay for it later), so it was like okay, what does that say? It says I have no power. I'm still struggling with being completely inconsequential in the world but also feeling like I have some sort of control. Because of course I know this whole thing, this whole disorder, is about trying to control the uncontrollable, scrambling around in the unknown for footing. What survival tools can I throw at this horrible shit to make myself feel safe. C was like, *what if you wished harm on me, like wished I had an aneurysm RIGHT NOW and I'll try to make myself have one too*, and I was like *holy shit, don't even say that*, and he said *yeah it felt really creepy saying it.* Then that's what I did. He said aneurysm or stroke or broken leg and I picked stroke because it'd be easier to repeat. I did some *Scanners* shit where I tried to make him have a stroke. I was saying *I hope you have a stroke right now, I want you to, I wish you would*, and he was saying it too, and he was telling me to really focus and try to make it happen, and we did it for a full five minutes, and it was wild, but he didn't have one. So we're breaking that link down more. I still have the urge to undo these things, but we do them so hard, repeat so much, that whatever ritual or neutralizing thing I'd need to do—I can't honestly even imagine what it could be. I'm screwed. It happened. It's done. Nothing I can do.

I moved onto groceries, and it was the same thing as yesterday, just this contaminated feeling of having bad hands, picturing little viruses crawling, wiggling, vibrating all over me. I touched my face, I touched my mouth. I put away all the groceries. I saved the brown bags when normally I'd recycle them. And now my hands are just AHHH, just filthy while I type this, but I can't wash them. I'm spreading it all over. But it's done.

It's done. I've touched/contaminated too much.

So the session was good again. Hard but good and I'm like *why is this good, why can I do this?* It's fucked. I fear happiness, so I'm waiting for when I fuck up.

Thursday, October 7, 2021

School was okay. I made this playlist of pop punk covers because I pitched this essay about them, so I was enjoying listening to that dumb shit on my commute. And class felt good because the time ticked by quickly, and the students seemed to get it, and I helped COVID-test-girl one-on-one after, and I wasn't afraid, really. I watched a little more of *Friday the 13th Part VI* when I got home before my session. This one's taking a long time to watch, I don't know why. It's the first one that gets kinda silly—where Tommy Jarvis is trying to burn Jason's dead body but ends up stabbing him in the chest with a rod from a cemetery gate, and then it starts storming and lightning strikes Jason and even though he's a decomposed corpse full of maggots he comes alive and kills Tommy's friend (who is Horshack), then goes to do the normal Jason stuff. But the best part is Tommy telling the cops, and he says *I tried to destroy him but I fucked up!!!* and it's my favorite line in the series so far. I'm typing most of this because there are a lot of triggering words in there about death, so I guess I'm just seeing if I can do it.

My session seemed way different today. We did a lot of planning, particularly around Jesse and Ezra, and how they play into my rituals and obsessions, like how I'm making them wash their hands, or not touch certain things. We made a plan to talk to them about stopping this and then about Jesse coming into a session for a little bit. We talked a lot about my brain and my questions regarding why the CBT is working, and when it will fail, and I felt very emotional about a lot of things, but the one that I can't shake is that C is very kind to me, and he seems genuinely absolutely psyched when I do well. It means so much. Sometimes when someone is that kind of nice, my heart can't really take it. I am always suspicious. But I think I'm accepting this, though it's hard. I wrote out a script detailing the path of my thinking about why I assume I'm gonna be extra crazy next week when Angus has a cancer scan. DUH it reminds me of my dad. I love my dog, but it's underlined hardcore with dad cancer stuff. The waiting, the unknown. So I wrote this script, said it out loud, and it felt bad. He told me to slow down and feel the emotions, and the end of the script is like *I did this and I'm a bad person, and I could've tried harder, and this is somehow my fault*, which is the core of it, that's why it's hard, me not doing the just-in-case rituals—*just in case this is affecting the universe in any way I might as well continue to do these elaborate rituals.* I was almost crying, and I felt just spent and bad, but also I was understanding it, the root of it. We moved on at the end to an exposure where I touched a package that had just come that day, which yeah, that shit sucks, but I did it, and I touched my face and mouth. I had the same feeling of bad hands, and I felt like the virus was on my clothes, but I kept them on and didn't wash my hands.

Friday, October 8, 2021

Started this day all fucked up. Woke up and attempted to get dressed with "bad" clothes, which ended up being tights that I haven't worn since my dad's funeral and a skirt and shirt I haven't worn in probably six years, but Jesse was trying to give Ezra a bath and he was acting like Jesse was murdering him (this is an exposure, me writing this), and he was screaming, and they were both screaming actually, and I tried to just stay in the moment and put on my clothes only one time without redoing it because "bad" stuff was happening, and then my shirt looked weird and I took it off, but the ponybead bracelet Ezra made for me got caught in the fabric and came undone, like completely exploded—the gimp was too brittle and it snapped— and the beads went everywhere. It was all this long line of things telling me *something bad will happen to him, he's the crying one, this broke, he will break, what could it be*, and I just stayed with it and got dressed, but he wouldn't stop being difficult, and I screamed and me screaming made me worse. Fucking chaos. It sounds so stupid written out, but it was a bad morning. The getting dressed exposure was hard. Ezra started crying at drop-off because he didn't want to go, didn't want me to leave, and so I was like *oh here's another sign*, and my brain's just this sinister fuck waiting for any excuse to launch into some bullshit reasoning, and OH it was my birthday HAHAHAHAHAHA.

On the way home I got some birthday texts, and one was from my dad's girlfriend, and I started crying because he's dead, she doesn't have to be nice to me, and the way she said good morning before wishing me a happy birthday just got me going. So I got home and I'm already an overflowing emotional mess, and Jesse gave me my present, which he had told me about, a vintage *Beavis and Butthead* shirt, and I'd been excited waiting for it, like *wow what a great find*, but he gave it to me, and we looked at it and fucking bitch that I am I said *are you sure this is vintage* and he looked at the mark and saw it was from 2017, and I was like *oh*, and he was like *I'm sorry*, and then me seeing him real-time realize he got duped was too much for me, and I felt bad I was disappointed, but I was, and I was sad he got fucked, and it was after that whole bad morning, and then he said he got me another present because he thought the shirt wasn't enough, and it was a pre-order of another t-shirt, and I lost it because he's gotten me a t-shirt every anniversary/birthday the past three times, and the *Beavis and Butthead* shirt thing had just happened, and again I am ungrateful, this is petty, but I lost it because I have so many shirts, and he keeps getting me more shirts and I have no room for the shirts and even if I did, I can't put them away because I have an elaborate ritual thing with them—laundry is a real weak spot for me. Conditions have to be ideal. Nothing iffy going on, no test results in limbo, no bad shit on the horizon, everyone in optimal health, quiet, peaceful atmosphere—all to fold clothes. I have to touch them a certain way, I have to hold my breath while doing it. I have to neutralize bad thoughts in my head. I just have too many fucking shirts, and I am a bitch. But this somehow balloons to like *here's my fucking wedding ring.* We've been together since we were fifteen. There's a lot of shit to draw from. We love each other but like, you know, everyone fights. And I feel like I'm under a lot of stress and pressure, and he's dealing with my nonsense.

But backing up, before I went really crazy, when I had only gone a little crazy, I went to get bagels with the intention of not cleaning the packaging before eating. The cemetery is right across from the bagel place so I went to the cemetery. I touched my dad's footstone, started talking to him. Last year he dropped off a coffee for my birthday. He'd started seriously declining around then, and it accelerated the following month. Most likely one of the last times he drove, and definitely one of the last times he drove to my house. I was fucked. I was just wrecked. I drove back with the bagels and I just—that's when we start the fight. We have to cut it short so I can go to therapy. My eyes are puffed up and I'm in a trance and when I get there I'm a little late because I still can't figure out the timing, and C asks me how I am, and I say a version of what happened, a lot less dumb detail. This time, when he asks the suicide question, I have to admit I said something like *maybe I just shouldn't be here anymore*, and it sucks to have to talk about those feelings. I went on about how maybe I'm sabotaging myself. Here's me getting all fucked up this morning, here's my brain fighting itself. We talked a lot, like a lot a lot. Then we moved on to an exposure: watching a video about how cancer forms in the body. I had to watch it four times, the last few times while performing tasks—cleaning my glasses, touching my phone, throwing something away. It was uncomfortable. But then we watched this video about cancer end-of-life shit, and it fucked me up. It was hard to watch. The woman died around Christmas, her skin was yellow, she was out of it—like stuff with my dad last year. It was rough. We ended it there. I'm glad. I know I have to watch this stuff, but it's like *A Clockwork Orange* a little bit.

Monday, October 11, 2021

Everyone in the house is sick. We're miserable. It's just a stupid thing, and I'm bouncing around thought-wise, *did I cause this by trying to get better and not doing safety rituals?* All weekend I was thinking about why this is working—we talked about it on Friday, me waiting for the other shoe to drop. The other part of my brain is scrambling to make me believe that the success I'm having now will lead to some mysterious, amorphous bunch of bad shit happening at some indeterminate date in the future. It's really wanting me to go with cancer, so it was like *HAHAHA have you felt your breast for lumps lately? Have you gone down that rabbit hole? What about Angus losing weight? Why is that happening? Google it now, look it up, ask people, find out information, do it do it DO IT.* The most acute anxiety thing was I gave Ezra a COVID test and had a complete meltdown while waiting the fifteen minutes. I know we have a cold, possibly two colds, ripping through us right now, but just introducing the idea of testing brought me to like a ninety on the scale and waiting for the result peaked at for sure a hundred, but it was negative. I couldn't do shit about it, just wait, so I was full-body shaking, crying, walking around in a daze. I'm traumatizing Ezra, I bet. I think of this constantly. I am 95% handling my shit in front of him, but that 5%, whoo boy. I try to explain worry and nervousness and anger, and I hope he understands. No one explained these things to me, so maybe it will help.

The weekend was full of worry. I'm taking a writing workshop with my friend Steven, and even on the Zoom call I couldn't focus. I was on my phone googling *dog chemo losing weight side effect* or some such thing, words in different orders. No reassurance provided. I was really looking forward to my session today because we hadn't yet talked too too much about why I do these reassurance-seeking behaviors, that whole thing. We talked about it, and he gave me a two-prong approach that made sense, the idea of first figuring out if there's a concrete step I can take, and if not (and probably if so, tbh) doing uncertainty exposure statements, like this one: *Angus may or may not have cancer,* that sort of thing. GOD I hate writing it. I hate thinking it. But he's got an ultrasound on Thursday, and I'm freaked out.

The big exposure I did today was…painting my nails, lol. It's another one of those "ideal conditions" activities that, if done wrong, could "infect" the future—if I fuck this up, then I will get bad news, something will go wrong, whatever. I'm locking in bad vibes. I'm carrying them into the future. So I'm in my office doing a Zoom and painting my nails while talking to C and walking him through everything, and I'm shaking while doing it because, again, I'm only choosing like the worst/hardest activities for me to do. I'm saying all sorts of bad things while doing this, and he's having me elaborate and explain what I mean when I say I feel bad, or bad stuff will happen—*well, what kind of bad stuff, what do you mean by bad?* God, it's anything and everything, but I was saying all these exposure statements about cancer and death and doing it, and I fucked up some of my nails, and did only three passes with the brush on some instead of four, or multiples of four. I would always do this and that's why my nails were always one goopy mess, and I'd have to remove all of it and start over, which is why it takes me like an hour to do, which is why I never do it or any sort of extra thing, why I'm just barely getting by, hygiene-wise, and so it was decidedly NOT ideal conditions, but I did it, and here I am typing with these nails, all black and smudged on the sides, leaving them, all the bad shit infused in them. I tried to do an uncertainty exposure statement a few hours after the session, and I started crying, so I don't know how good I'm going to be at that. All I can do is keep trying because the anxiety has no place to go. C did tell me this really good metaphor of what I should be doing. "Driving the bus." Like I'm driving the bus to someplace that's consistent with my values and morals, I forget what he said, but I'm driving it, and I can't help who comes onto the bus, but I can help how much I engage with them. So all these bad ideas and thoughts keep hopping on, and I've just got to learn how to co-exist. It makes a lot of sense to me, but now I've just got to really put it into practice.

Tuesday, October 12, 2021

Same little library room at school. I was able to stay away from everyone. Jesse came to the beginning of my session, and we talked about making a plan for him to help me, specifically what to do when I'm reassurance-seeking. I was nervous about him being in this little space, where I do all this work he knows nothing about. Everything went okay, except I got embarrassed when he said something to C about me being smart. I feel dumb in general, especially for these things I do, these things I believe, the space they take up in my brain. Maybe when I have a clear head, or maybe when I learn to be okay with the chaos that's there, things will be different. The rest of the session I worked on repeating uncertainty exposure statements, which has been the most difficult task for me so far. *Angus could have cancer or he could not have cancer—I don't know—there's no way to know for sure right now—there's nothing I can do about it.* No control, no answers, flailing in the dark. I don't know how other people stand it.

———

Later, everything turned awful because we got an email saying a kid tested positive at Ezra's school. I'll spare details here because all I do is run the numbers and the exposure timetable and the test timetable and the Google results over in my mind, and it's making me feel sick. I gave him an at-home rapid test, waited the fifteen minutes. I was calmer, although I checked the test more frequently, but what can I do? It was negative. What can I do? During all of it, I had what I guess looking back now would be considered some sort of breakthrough. I felt like I had to make a decision—okay, all this shit is happening, so do I go back and do rituals? Was CBT the wrong decision? Or do I keep going. I decided to keep going. I'm not sure of my reasons, though I suspect deep down I feel like I'd hate myself (more) if I gave up, and I am understanding more and more the lack of connections between events. So I'm just blindly accepting the therapy now, like okay, I'll give it one last go. I signed Ezra up for a PCR test at Rite Aid because CVS was booked, so I have to wait for that, and Angus's scan is Thursday. That could make or break me.

This is what C suggested I use for when I'm asking Jesse for reassurance. He's supposed to say something like: *I hear you that this is really scary. My understanding of how I can support you is to not provide reassurance here. I know that may be pretty hard for you, and I believe in you that you can handle it. And I'm happy to support you in other ways that don't involve reassurance or doing rituals.*

I'm supposed to think: *Is there an answer that would be satisfying? Does the other person have information I don't? Am I not trusting my own eyes? Have I already asked this?* The answers are usually no, no, yes, yes. I didn't get a chance to go over it with Jesse because of all the bullshit going on, but I hope we can. I hope it will be useful.

Wednesday, October 13, 2021

I woke up at 5am and went on Reddit to learn about how long Rite-Aid PCR tests take and found out a) a long time, and b) they can come back inconclusive. I made a rapid test appointment at CVS for today and a PCR there for tomorrow. CVS canceled the rapid. I couldn't go back to sleep. I tried to picture myself driving the bus, all the thoughts just fucked-up passengers, but they were too loud. I got up and talked to Jesse, and he was like *why don't you just take him to the doctor*. I knew they'd just do a PCR and it'd take over two days and I needed faster answers, but then I figured maybe I was being a horrible mother not taking him. Maybe he has bronchitis or pneumonia or an infection.

I called and got him in at 9:30. Lungs looked good. They did a PCR, results in forty eight hours. This stuff is so technical and boring. My brain is non-stop, but I don't want to think about tests all day. I want to have ideas or something, you know? After the doctor, I took him to the cool coffee place downtown with the skeletons and creepy clown and he loved it. Even then, I was like why am I bringing him around, he's this bomb of contagion. I did the rapid last night and it was negative. But did I swirl it around in his nose enough? Is it accurate? I canceled the Rite-Aid and CVS tests. I'd been emailing with C, so he knew I was going through it.

I gave him the whole story during our session. He was probably bored, too. But he said a good exposure would be to call the school to see if Ezra could come back, because I'm scared to have him go back. The school said they hadn't been specific last night, but they weren't accepting home tests, and it was weird that a PCR was going to take so long (it's not weird?) and I could try this other place. C had me call there, and I'm going at nine tomorrow. They "want them in school" like yeah, I guess me too. Doing the best I can.

We worked on exposure stuff the rest of the time. I folded Ezra's laundry. It's been sitting out all crumpled in a basket since July or August. I had to say *COVID* while doing it, which felt like I was infecting the clothing. Like summoning it. I want to erase those sentences, but I won't. I had to say this, another uncertainty exposure statement: *The test could be positive or it could be negative, but I can't know right now—I have to wait—and if it's positive, he's in danger, I put him in danger, he might die, we might die, other children might die, and I'm a bad mom for sending him to school in the first place.* He said that's the root of a lot of these things—guilt, shame, all that. It feels awful. It's a pit inside. I put Ezra to bed and we bumped into each other in the dark because he was fucking around, and it hurt my skull, and I immediately started crying, and I couldn't stop, but I kept it quiet, and he fell asleep, and I kept crying. I'm truly starting to understand that I have no real control. It's scary. Nothing I do, no behavior I have, has any bearing on anything. I've been believing differently since I was six years old—it's really been that long now that I think about it, when I'd obsess about finding tumors on my body. When I was worried everyone around me was going to die. Not, like, eventually. Immediately, and horribly. I don't know. It's a lot to take in.

Thursday, October 14, 2021

Today all the things I was worried about worked themselves out. This is helping to prove that my behavior has little to do with the outcomes. My rituals don't protect me. The way I'm thinking has shifted radically, and I'm unsure how to go forward. This is all new. My OCD brain is scattered and desperate, trying to punch holes in everything still, and I think it will do that forever, so I just have to come back to that "driving the bus" thing. The thoughts are there in the background. C said it's like a dog. You have to let it bark.

So, yeah. I played I Spy while waiting for the in-person rapid test results. They were negative. I felt relief for about two hours, and then, ah yes, Angus was still at the vet getting a battery of tests. Around one we got good news about him—the cancer hasn't spread. There may be evidence it's not there at all? I don't know because I didn't reassurance-seek. I took everything at face value. Wow, look at me. While I was waiting, I again made the "good" choice of resisting rituals and OCD behavior, and I cleaned up the office. It didn't matter that I touched things wrong or looked at things wrong. I was like, here's the test, if it's good news, then definitely no connection. The news was still good. I feel like I'm starting to get it. C and I talked mostly about how I'm afraid to say that things are going well. I did an exposure around it. I said *I'm happy, things are good right now, I'm doing well in treatment, and I'm excited for the future* for like ten minutes. The anxiety was highest right before—I couldn't even say it. It peaked and went down then spiked again, but it eventually stayed at like a seventy-five. We talked about take-home messages, and I told him I was understanding things in a whole new light and felt like I was on drugs. What is being happy all about? Can I even think about it? I don't know.

Here's some of what I was saying: *Fighting the anxiety never actually worked in the way that I was intending it to work... I would end up getting extremely frustrated, and the anxiety wouldn't go away, it would just come back. I was creating all these rules and they don't make logical sense. Fighting the anxiety led to me being unhappy.* I was also saying something like: *The very idea of being happy or enjoying life was tied to engaging in safety behaviors. I was trying to achieve happiness by avoiding danger. I was trying to avoid bad things, and they still happened. Happiness never actually entered the equation.*

Almost immediately after I repeated these phrases, I got another email about another COVID exposure, this time on Tuesday. I made a test appointment for Sunday, but I couldn't sleep. I woke up again at 5am, nauseated with a racing heart.

After I found out, I emailed C to tell him I should probably do a virtual appointment and he said back: *I can absolutely see how that would be a bummer (and at the same time receiving some bad news sometimes is unavoidable!). Good luck tonight! I know you have your work cut out for you. For what it's worth, you're doing great. Life will continue to happen.* I keep re-reading the email, repeating it in my head. I don't know. I mentioned this before, but the idea that someone else is invested in my success feels so nice and kind that I am having a hard time dealing with it. And life continuing to happen. Yeah. The temptation to ritualize has been strong, and I'm trying hard to resist.

Friday, October 15, 2021

Was up at 5am again, got some work done. I guess that's nice. I couldn't sleep after that though, and I am exhausted. I presented to a Brazilian college class virtually on creative writing for an hour and a half in the morning, and it ended up being so much fun that it distracted me for a bit. Talking about myself like I'm successful or like I know anything at all lolol. But it was cool. I bounced from worry to worry the rest of the day. I wasn't able to resist little "checking" behaviors like before. I asked Jesse over and over if he thought Ezra was going to be okay, if he'd be feeling some symptom by now. I asked Ezra if anyone had been coughing a lot at school. Who was the most disgusting kid? And did that kid happen to sit with him at lunch? As if narrowing down who was the positive case would somehow allow me to calculate our odds while we waited out the next couple of incubation days. I felt guilty and bad for the checking. Like I had a choice and made the wrong one; in the past I honestly didn't feel like I even had a choice—I had to do the behaviors. I only googled once,

but I felt like shit after. I felt the extreme urge to ritualize. Like hardcore URGE, this pull, and I resisted but
barely, just forced myself, which also didn't feel totally
healthy because I wasn't really riding the wave of anxiety, but God I'm so fucked up today. Took Ezra to get
donuts, took a picture of the donuts, but only once. It
didn't feel like THE picture, didn't feel right, bad
thoughts while I clicked the shutter, etc. etc. but…I left
it. Didn't delete. I'm trying to focus on these little wins.

At my appointment, we worked on a plan for when
these "speed bumps" happen. When some unwanted
thing occurs and I'm losing it. Some trigger. Whatever.
I know most of what I'm supposed to do now, the signs
I have to be on the lookout for: initial panic, worry,
trouble sleeping, urges to perform rituals and seek reassurance. When that shit happens, I need to do an exposure, or an exposure statement. Or I need to reach
out for help, which is not the same thing as reassurance-
seeking because you're not asking for answers, just support, like *here is my plan, will you support me?* And I have
to keep in mind the difference between a slip and a full-
blown relapse, the difference between an urge and a
choice. C also said to try to create a character around
the OCD "voice" that pulls me, and from what I de-
scribed, he said it sounded like the bad guy in a
1980s/90s anti-drug commercial, the guy in the alley-
way. It's definitely some bad dude in my head.

Oh to reiterate, or maybe I didn't even say, I was totally fucked up coming in. On the verge of tears. Worry-hopping, spiraling, sad, TERRIFIED. Once we made the plan, which took like an hour, I started to feel like I wasn't freefalling. Like I jumped out of an airplane with no parachute. Because now we built the parachute. Then we did an exposure statement: *My son was exposed to COVID, so he might have COVID, and if he has it, he could die, and I can't fully control if that happens. That would mean I've failed as a mother, and I don't think I could survive that. I could have a breakdown or attempt suicide. The aftermath is unknown.* I had to really pay attention to *I can't fully control if that happens* and *the aftermath is unknown.* Scary shit. I felt really anxious at first, but it started to dissipate, then turned into terror and sadness, because I was picturing Ezra dead, little kid in a casket, so I started crying, but then eventually I sat with it, kept saying it, and it got replaced with this calm feeling of just being bummed out, and he said *yeah that makes sense, that's the feeling that usually happens.* I'd rather be calm and clear-headed and sad than anxious and a complete maniac. I'm going to try to do this this weekend. My homework is also to resist testing Ezra before Sunday. Just got really grossed-out typing all of this. FUCK IT FUCK THIS AHHHH

Cried again while putting Ez to bed. Did Reiki on him and he said *Reiki is fake!!!* But then he let me. Then I did it on myself and that's when I cried. I saw a medium last night and she told me to keep up with the healing and that animals will be my niche. She also told me my dad was the one leaving feathers everywhere (we keep finding feathers everywhere; I did not tell her this) and that my dad was talking about coffee (that last "conversation" I "had" with him—me talking to his footstone—was about coffee) and she couldn't have known this either but I dyed my hair from neon purple to reddish brown (normal), and she said my dad was saying he liked my hair, that "that's [his] Em." I felt sad but also nice but mostly sad. I'm still sad, but I'm going to let the emotions come and go, see what happens. Also I am going to have a beer, just one beer, a perfectly innocuous beer. I feel guilty but also I am unsure of other ways to unwind. Maybe we can talk about that.

Monday, October 18, 2021

I'm not really sure how I was able to keep anxiety down this weekend. If I think too hard it might feed the anxiety, might create little blips, little red flags where I'd need to investigate and narrate around them. That's what I've been noticing—the need to narrate, to create stories and connections. *Have you thought of this and then this happening, which could only happen because you did this or that...* on and on. I'm learning to exhale at certain times—the ends of pages while I'm reading, the ends of songs. I had this previous narration that exhaling was like the final exhale, the final breath, so: death, and if I exhale in the wrong spot I'm fucking something up and it will infect the night or day after I put down the book or finish the song, so I need to reread and restart the track. I also can't end on words related to death—*death, dying, dead, breathing, breath, breathe*, I could go on. The narration used to play out in front of me, hyper-speed, but now it's habitual. There's not even much of a narration anymore, just this "weird thing I have to do" that I can't help but do. I'm becoming aware of my control over these vestigial ritual behaviors, the ones that feel like habits. Anyway, I went off track here. The weekend was fine. I took it hour-by-hour, re-frained/restrained myself from testing Ez with the home kit. It was reassuring that he seemed to have no symp-toms. I felt sad on Friday night after my session. I felt sad on and off Saturday too. I'm sitting with sadness, seeing where it goes. Sunday was okay, but I took Ez for the PCR they wanted him to take for school. Then we bought tie-dye shirts at the dwindling farmer's market.

Woke up early because I told C I'd take a test before coming. I put too much of the liquid in the test because I wasn't awake all the way, and I think it made the test look unreliable—I checked it literally every minute, watched it turn pink, called Jesse at one point because he was getting coffee and gas and I shouldn't have let him leave me. But it was fine, it was negative. I took a picture and sent it: reassurance-seeking, mhmm. Bad this morning. Then some guilt, duh. I got to my ap-pointment early, which hasn't happened before. We talked about the weekend, and then a little about what other things I wanted to cover before treatment ends, which honestly still sends me into a panic, or not panic, like a sadness. I think there's sadness under all my panic. Attempts to avoid sadness. I'm putting in all this work on myself, carving out the time, and now it's almost over. I have a doctor who is really working hard, really wanting me to succeed (not saying my others didn't or don't, but the vibe is different), and soon I'll be off on my own. I keep bringing it up. There's no solution, idk.

I watched the original cancer video, and I was largely okay, just little anxiety spikes around specific words and phrases. Then I watched the end-of-life one twice, and it fucked me up, but C said it's like normal-people sad too, which I guess helps me understand that the feelings aren't incorrect or totally out of proportion. We had this long conversation about me saying/admitting I was happy and how terrifying it is for me, and I ended up going pretty deep into what I think is the root of this, which is that I was raised Catholic (lol). I am all entangled with guilt. I was in second or third grade, standing in line, trying to catalogue my sins to tell some old guy in the hallway, and I could never come up with enough (because uhhh I was a kid), so I'd exaggerate some, which meant I could use lying as one too, and I think it got all warped in my mind that any time I experienced fun or pleasure, I was doing something wrong. Lots of things reinforced this throughout my life. I had the added element of being a Very Bad Teen, which I am still answering for in my adult life. I am all about this magical balance of power, this good and evil, this *I have sinned and now I must pay*. It was a good, useful conversation. I worked on some exposures surrounding this, making statements like *I am looking forward to this* without couching it in a bigger negative statement. We had a lot of other things on the list, so I plan on working hard tomorrow. Have I mentioned writing this feels extremely dumb and embarrassing? Because it does. Oh, and Ezra's PCR was negative, so I feel better about coming in person, but it means he's got to go back to school, back to that cesspool. Cool times! Bye!

Tuesday, October 19, 2021

School was okay today even though I was calling them up one by one to talk about their methodology plans for their research projects, and that meant they were right there in my face. I've never realized how many people are close talkers, or maybe it's normal and my sense of the way people used to talk will forever be off now. But most of it was fine.

During session today, we spent an hour and a half (I apologized after and C said apology not accepted) talking about what therapy looks like for me after this. The biggest shift in me thinking about this is that I had assumed I should always be in therapy. Like *I am sick, I need help.* But after our talk today, I'm thinking maybe short-term, goal-oriented therapy is more effective for me. EMDR worked, CBT is working. Talking about my bullshit since 2002 has... not worked. Almost twenty years of this stuff. There were a lot of times where I was just fucking around, not really trying to get better or understand what was happening with me, just expecting to be fed a pill and be fixed. But I finally feel like I'm gaining control over my own mind. I'm re-thinking all of this. At one point, C said he enjoys talking with me, and that was incredibly validating, which made me feel pathetic, that my urge to be liked is too strong. But I've spent a lot of time bouncing back and forth between doctors, psych and regular, and some have made me feel okay, but I think that's why I'm having a hard time with this ending. It's making me rethink the whole idea of being in therapy and what I want to get out of it—what are my goals? They should be right there when I go in for an appointment. I need to be better about self-advocacy. But I entered therapy when I was fourteen or fifteen, and it was my mom bringing me in like *help me she won't go to school what do I do*, so I was being forced into it, then DCF got involved after my assault, then going to the hospital and being put on all these medications, and I just grew up in it. Now it's like, how can I use this tool to actually give me a better life? What does that even look like?

I painted my nails watching the end-of-life video today. The difficulty was ninety-five. Locking in cancer-talk, bad vibes, bleh...hated it. I felt sad, terrified. All the little triggering parts of the video, the dying woman's slow, slurred speech, the way she pulls the caretaker's hand onto her own arm, just to be touched. I started thinking about how I brought lotion to my dad in hospice and massaged his arms and hands and legs. How thin his skin was, how papery. I let the thought linger, the sadness fill. My homework is to do the second coat, and then to not seek reassurance surrounding Ez going back to school.

Wednesday, October 20, 2021

I felt pretty anxious today because it was Ezra's first day back at school, but I resisted going over and over *please wear your mask please for the love of God* type stuff with him. My big task today was going to Target because I hadn't been in a bit, and it presented me with challenges I'd constantly failed at in the past. I have always had a hard time picking out items, and often if the situation is not ideal before touching the item, and I touch it, if something gets bad or fucked up—some outside influence, the wrong finger touching, or if someone is coughing/screaming/crying, or I hear a triggering word in a song/have a bad feeling or thought in my head, I will have to redo. Put down, pick a new one. If it's the last one left, oh well, guess I'm not buying that today. Two items today that had issues were Ezra's toothpaste (that good blue sparkle Crest kind, not that it matters, but it was my first time getting it since I was a kid) and a package of socks for him. The socks just felt not meant to be. But I put them in the cart and felt anxious, got pangs, but I did it. And the toothpaste, well, a lady had a coughing fit in the aisle while I was getting it, so that's somehow infecting me/the toothpaste, and I would normally put it back, wait until she left, and then pick a different one. But today I just put it in the cart. I didn't clean anything off when I got home, a bit of anxiety floating around, but it went down, came back, etc. But it did go down, and that's a good sign.

Today we did an exposure based around my fear of Ezra dying. I went over the list of disturbing images that come into my brain, the main ones—COVID and cancer, then murder, and I didn't mention specifically school shootings but that too, and any sort of accident that could kill him. My brain shows me him dead and bloody, head caved in and gaping, or dead in a casket, pale, ashen rings around his eyes, dead in so many ways (I hate typing this). I'm reading my script and all this shit is going on, all these thoughts streaming in. I started to feel just really sad about the whole thing, which was what the anxiety was masking. Then C asked me about how my emotions were treated when I was a child, like what my emotional life was like. I said I was a super sensitive kid who got sad about inanimate objects breaking like they were hurt and had feelings, and I kept broken crayons and popped balloons, and I felt everything, and I cried a lot, and there were times I remember feeling scared and sad and watching the sun set out my window, and I missed my mom all the time, even when she was there. Sounds so fucking dramatic, but I remember this sharp fear running through me. I stopped going to school when I was around fourteen, and that turned out to have pretty bad consequences: school said I could go on homebound but I'd need to quit my gifted program. My boyfriend broke up with me when I was in the hospital. My friends didn't understand and got mad if I didn't feel up to hanging out. My mom couldn't handle how I was feeling (not her fault; she didn't know what to do), my sisters were upset and traumatized, my dad didn't believe in whatever was wrong with me. I was sad for like three solid years, and it was bad too—sex and fighting and rage blackouts and self-harm and missing school. In college I was like *okay this hasn't gotten me anywhere and people are actively leaving my life so let me work my ass off and get a 4.0 and then that'll show everyone and also erase all of the bad stuff, and I won't be sad anymore.* Surprise, that didn't work in the way I thought, and instead the anxiety parts still lingered and got stronger. People still bring up how fucked up I was at fifteen, and I'm thirty-four. I was having a hard time today in the session because I've tried to not be sad for so long. And here it comes. Here it comes.

Oh, and I took Ezra to Spirit Halloween which is his first big store since March 2020, so that was a big risk after exploring everything in that exposure. Today was a lot, and I'm feeling it. C said to do something soothing tonight, so I'm going to shower now and be alone.

And sad! Which is okay. I told C it's starting to feel like I'm graduating.

Thursday, October 21, 2021

I didn't get too much time to reflect on what C and I discussed last meeting, but I did tell Jesse about it. Honestly, I don't even really know if I'm supposed to reflect on it. Maybe I'm just supposed to purely feel. It's been this oddly welcome feeling, and that seems wrong, but I won't judge it. I did all the things I had to do today, everything sadness-tinged. School was fine. I cut it short because there wasn't too much I had to tell the students today. I thought I'd do this reflecting thing on my drive, but instead I was in a daze listening to music and driving, getting from here to there. It's weird because the sadness feels unattached to a thought or event, like I am sad because of the exposure statement I had to read, the real bummer one I wrote yesterday about Ezra dying and me burying him, but I'm also sad, almost a more palpable, on-the-verge-of-tears kind of sad, about treatment ending tomorrow. I was able to have three solid weeks to tackle something that's been part of me for so long. Maybe I'm sad that I'm happy. How dumb is that. Maybe I'm sad because I can let go of these behaviors. Maybe I'm just fucking sad. It's like they have books and pretty much a whole movement nowadays for kids to feel their feelings, like more extreme than Mr. Rogers stuff, like *oh wow I can see you're having big feelings and it's okay to have them.* That's what I feel like. Maybe I need to be treated like a child who doesn't yet understand how to manage and control. I have to ask C tomorrow what the behaviors were protecting me from—being anxious or being sad? Or was the anxiety protecting me from being sad? Before, it seemed like a big convoluted mess of bad, and now it's got these connections and layers. This sadness feels huge, but it's almost an ache, not a sharp thing, this dull, muted feeling.

I went into my session today like that and let C know I wasn't really able to devote space to myself. I did mention I was able to resist certain rituals/compulsions, like "missing" some landmark on my commute. In the past, I'd set certain goals like *oh I have to make sure I see Ezra's school or look at certain words on a sign* and if I missed doing it, I'd turn around and re-drive the little stretch. So that happened today but I didn't drive back. I'm noticing more and more these other little things I do that are OCD behaviors that don't happen every day but are clearly something I need to address. For an exposure today I watched some videos on children and COVID, and they had a lot of triggering words in them, and the images sucked, blurred-out faces of kids in hospital beds, all scrunched up on the big mattresses. They were news videos so they used scare tactics and it was so loud, even when I turned the volume down finally. Ezra got home about an hour into the session, and he got a Lego Michael Meyers minifigure in the mail and was losing his mind running around excited, so I kept having to shush him and couldn't focus. I felt like I wasn't focused at all this session to be honest, which made me a little mad because it's the second to last one. I was worried I was forgetting something to cover with C and I'd have stuff lingering after our session tomorrow.

The big exposure I did today was an overcorrection—watching and listening to these videos while folding Ezra's clothes. The anxiety would not go down. I was getting a little frustrated because Ezra was loud again, and I was trying to work, and the anxiety wouldn't budge, but then C said maybe it wouldn't, and I'd have to learn how to do the task with the anxiety there. So I did. After, I said I was going to take a walk because I felt totally wiped. He encouraged me to make space for things like that, so I'll try to incorporate it more. I walked around the block, kind of blank-headed, all feeling. Sometimes I get caught up that this is the same world, same planet, that it was when I was a kid. Same trees, this same house. I still feel the same as always about a late October day that's too hot. How orange, how golden.

———

Maybe I should get myself a cake.

Friday, October 22, 2021

Okay, I did it. I feel really weird.

I went out in the morning to get werewolf fur for Ezra's costume at Joann Fabrics. Got coffee. Signed up for a booster shot. All good things, little good things. Jesse and I started getting all nostalgic for our city in the 90s, as we do, trying to figure out where the Joann Fabrics near us used to be before it moved to Wolcott Street, before it closed down for good, and then arguing about it but like, nice arguing. We're in a better spot. We kind of get everything out there and then are normal again. Trying again, fixing whatever was wrong. We called my mom for her opinion and started talking about JayMar and Fascia's Chocolate and the vacuum repair shop. It's my favorite activity, just remembering how things used to be. So many things are good in my memory. So many things are better than they actually were. Then I watched an episode of *Intervention* and got ready to leave. I was on my way and C called and said he needed

to meet virtually, which was good because then I would-
n't hit rush hour. We spent about an hour talking about
self-compassion. I was sort of like *yeah, sure, I'll figure it
out* and he called me out a little bit, and he's right because I won't do any of it. So we talked more concretely
about these things. I'm still sad, so we talked more about
that, and he told me this term backdraft. He said it
happens to some people when they start practicing self-
compassion. The pain at first increases because the old
pain has to come out, kind of like opening a door to a
burning room. He asked me to think of a time when I
was comforted, how I would like to be comforted, and
how I would comfort someone else. I was drawing
blanks. I don't know how I want to be comforted. I was
hugged after I was assaulted, so not hugs. I will occa-
sionally ask to hug someone, but my arms on the outside, no being enveloped. I will stroke my own hair
sometimes, rub my own shoulders. These are pathetic
things, but I do them. They're comforting. I can do
Reiki on myself, which I was reminded of when C suggested an exercise—putting my hand on my chest and
feeling the sensation. That's basically energy work. And
then comforting someone else? I don't know, man. If
someone is crying around me I am sort of like *get me
out of here.* These are things I have to think about more.
We came up with a tentative plan to be intentional
about activities I'm already doing, like making myself
coffee or tea and being, I don't know, fully present and
aware of it as a self-care act, which I know is all trendy
and overblown commercially, but I am fucked up, so it

makes sense. I told C I'll do a calm movie night tonight with lights and candles. The movie is *Wes Craven's New Nightmare* though.

We moved on to exposures. The first was to watch cancer drug ads and fold clothes, and I hastily searched Keytruda (I hate typing this word! So many of these words!), which was the drug my dad was almost going to go on but then he was too sick—nothing was going to work. I pressed play and I was sharing my screen and listening to the ad but not watching, and C was like *wait this isn't a real ad*, and it was actually just the audio of a Keytruda ad but someone had stitched together *Breaking Bad* clips? And he said *yeah I was like wow that guy really looks like Bryan Cranston*, and it was funny but embarrassing because I'm an idiot for not noticing but I was so nervous about doing it that I couldn't even bear to look at the screen. I just heard the audio and winced and focused on folding the shirts. This was not what I should've been doing, so I deserved the embarrassment, to kind of wake myself up.

For the next one I did a breast cancer ad, which was three million times harder. I watched it, and I had to sit down because I was so shaky and holding my breath the whole time. My mind was spiraling. We stopped because the session was almost done. I kind of hated stopping because I thought the last one we'd do would be a nice, complete rise-and-fall anxiety situation, a good exposure. But it was too hard. I imagine this will happen a lot, and that I'll need to get used to it, and get used to being alone, without C, when it happens. Then he said all this really nice stuff about how impressive what I'm doing is and how he couldn't figure out how my level of distress wasn't matching up to my outward display, but how everything makes sense now, and how (I think?) it was impressive that I kind of took the severity of my OCD, the immense time and energy I "put into" ritualizing etc. and put it into going hardcore in the other direction, and he said he was glad to be a part of this. I don't have any kind of adequate words to describe how much that meant to me, that whole part where he was saying nice stuff—I tried, I said thank you, I said that I've never had success before and was grateful, but he was kind of like, *I didn't really do anything but implement the program* or whatever, which is not really true in my opinion. I could've failed if I got the sense the other person didn't genuinely care about my success. I have to believe he must have. I think if I'm successful it must be good for him, too, so I have to believe he would care. Or does care. Maybe people care about me? Maybe I am starting to care about myself? I'm going to see him every other week, and in the in-between weeks I'll be doing my own session structured similarly where I'd check in and then practice an exposure.

When I hung up, I was still that same on-and-off sad. I went to make tea. I did it slowly. I boiled the water. I poured the water in the mug. I opened the package, slipped the bag into the water. While it was steeping I sat and cried. Then I pulled out the bag, sopping, and dangled it over my open palm so I could feel the droplets burn my skin. I cried more. When I was done, I took my tea outside. The air was so cool. It was golden still, and I could breathe.

March 2022

Yesterday I got rear-ended while stopped at a blinking red. I've been awake for a week so I assumed it was my fault. It was just me and Ezra in the car, coming home from Dollar Tree. I tried to be somewhat normal and reassuring to him although I was dazed and my brain was playing catch-up. A man wearing a cowboy hat witnessed the whole thing, asked if everyone was okay, if he should call the cops. He was smoking the tiny stub of a cigarette. The other driver came out of his car and shook his head. I turned off my car, called the cops. I walked to my trunk to assess damage—minimal for me, but his car was totally fucked. Accordioned front, smashed lights, glass all over. When he saw me look at his car he started yelling, only there was something wrong with his speech, something muffled and unclear. I couldn't understand much except all the *fucks* and the seething and the immediate threat of violence. My mind went sort of blank and I started arguing back, like *dude what the fuck, you crashed into me, it's a red light*, the adrenaline weird inside me. I couldn't understand what he was saying. Then I remembered Ezra, so I climbed into the passenger seat and locked the doors.

A cop came so I got out again, license and registration in shaking hands. The driver started screaming at the cop, and the cop told the driver to get back into his car. I hid by Ezra's rolled-up window, peeked around my SUV to watch. The cowboy came over to me and said not to worry, that I didn't do anything wrong. I felt tears coming. I said the driver was scaring my son. As I said it, I realized I was also scaring my son. The cowboy waved at Ezra and said *everything's okay buddy, your mommy didn't do anything.* I thought, fuck, it should've been me saying something like that.

The cop was sorting through our insurance papers and trying to talk to the driver. The cowboy brought up the driver's speech to me, said it sounded like he'd had a stroke. He said he should know, because he himself had had multiple strokes. I started asking him about his strokes. He told me about arteries and surgeries and how it was only a matter of time before another one killed him. I said I was so sorry to hear that. He said *that's life.* I didn't know what to say after that, so I thanked him and said I was lucky he witnessed the accident. He told me he was just crossing over to the Rite-Aid for cat food. I started asking him about his cats when the cop came back over. The driver peeled out. The cop said *he's in the wrong, not you.* I felt the adrenaline still charging. The cowboy said if I needed him, I could find him at Mike's Pizza downtown. He sits at the tables there, watching his son make pizzas all day.

I'm writing this because, one, it's full of words that would've set me off six months ago, and also because: nothing I did or didn't do (besides stopping at the red light) caused this car accident or allowed it to be less serious than it could've been. Talking about strokes will not cause me to have a stroke or this man to have another one. Taking Ezra out in public had nothing to do with the crash. Listening to a particular song had nothing to do with it. Wearing a particular outfit had nothing to do with it. Having one or two moments of joy in my life had nothing to do with it. Getting "better," as they say, had nothing to do with it. Cowboy man, yes, you're right. That's life.

When I finished CBT, I'd merely chipped away the top layer of bullshit. Rituals and safety behaviors covering up sadness and fear. But that first layer—I'll give myself some credit—felt impenetrable. It had adhered so permanently onto these other things that I'd never been able to address them. Now I'm addressing them. They're manifesting in strange ways—immense sadness, fear of sleep, nocturnal panic attacks, hypnic jerks, insomnia, terror, palpitations, severe hypochondria.

All that said, it's manageable. It feels awful, but I keep thinking of that Molly Brodak poem: "The amount of fear/I am ok with/is insane."

My body has reached its limit. There's nowhere for it to go. I have to be okay with fear. I have to be okay.

Yesterday I got in that car accident, and the coursing adrenaline protected me from feeling any pain. Now it's worn off. My neck hurts when I look up or turn my head, my swollen muscles and ribs ache, and my lower back feels pinched. Whatever protective thing my body was doing is cleared and the pain is free to come coursing in, and only now can I truly assess the damage.

Acknowledgements

Thank you to Jesse and Ezra. Thank you to C and my other doctors. Thank you to my mom, to the rest of my family, my friends, my Internet friends, to Tim Parrish, Jessica Forcier, my SCSU MFA and FYE families, Steven Arcieri for helping with the start of this, Aaron Burch for publishing my first OCD thing, Elle Nash and the TEXTURES crew for being all-around great people, Michael Wheaton and Autofocus, Caroline Fernandes, Alex Capaldo, Lauren Mancuso, Kayleigh Mierzejewski, and Donna Ring. Oh, and thank you to the cowboy.

About the Author

Emily Costa's work can be found in *X-R-A-Y, Hobart, Barrelhouse, Wigleaf,* and elsewhere. She is currently working on a novel sort of about her father's video store, as well as a book of short stories. You can follow her on Twitter @emilylauracosta.

Scan for supplemental book content

[a]

Made in the USA
Columbia, SC
01 June 2022

61163512R00057